The XXL Keto Diet Book for UK

Quick and Delicious Recipes for Every Day incl. 14 Days Keto Challenge for Longterm Weight Loss

Food Club UK

ISBN - 9798717374682

Table of Contents

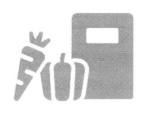

Introduction

What is the Keto Diet?

Widely known as 'Keto,' the ketogenic diet is a healthy eating plan that consists of low-carbohydrate, moderate-protein, and high-fat foods. Through the increased consumption of fat and drastically reduced intake of carbs, the body is forced to enter a metabolic state called ketosis where fat is transformed into ketones in the liver.

In ketosis, the body stops using carbohydrates as its primary energy source and instead burns fat. This leads to a variety of health benefits including reduced blood sugar, lower cholesterol levels, and quick weight loss.

By turning fat into ketones, the body and brain are supplied with a new source of energy. And when done right, this can enhance health in ways that are nearly impossible to achieve with most other forms of dieting.

Why the Keto Diet?

Even with countless diet plans to choose from, the Keto Diet remains one of the most popular throughout the world – and it's no wonder why. Studies have shown that the ketogenic diet is far more effective than a low-fat diet at maintaining weight loss in the long term.

However, unknown to many, its benefits extend even further than this. Aside from incredible weight loss results, Keto dieters have also reported:

- Increased energy levels.

- Improved acne and skin health.

- Regulated blood sugar levels.

- Lowered 'bad' cholesterol and improved healthy cholesterol.

- Stronger focus and mental clarity.

- Staying full for longer and reduced cravings.

- Decreased blood pressure in overweight individuals.

- Better control over epileptic symptoms in both children and adults.

It should be noted that all new keto dieters are expected to experience tiredness when their bodies first enter ketosis, but once the body adjusts, these health benefits are quickly and easily gained.

Rules of the Ketogenic Diet

Low Amounts of Net Carbohydrates

Net carbohydrates can be calculated by subtracting the amount of fibre and sugar alcohols from the 'Total Carbohydrates' number on the nutrition label. To enter a state of ketosis, make sure that your intake of net carbohydrates does not exceed 50g a day. And for the most success, try to stay below 20g.

In order for the ketogenic diet to work, it's crucial that your intake of net carbohydrates is heavily managed. This means paying attention to the nutrition labels on your groceries and staying away from many often-used foods such as pasta, potatoes, and bread. Keep in mind that starchy vegetables such as peas and corn are also off-limits during the keto diet.

Moderate Amounts of Protein

Protein is vital for maintaining your body's proper function and keeping the body lean. Low-carb seafood, poultry, and red meat are encouraged on the keto diet for all who eat meat, though they should always be secondary to the fatty foods on your plate.

Too much protein can prevent the body from entering ketosis, so make sure to keep your meals varied. Furthermore, always choose fattier cuts of meat over any lean alternatives.

High Amounts of Fat

Fat is your friend on the ketogenic diet. This means embracing many delicious high-fat foods that other diets restrict such as butter, cheese, cream, olive oil, and avocado. Dieters are conditioned to fear the fat content in foods, but the keto diet thrives when these numbers are high as long as the other macros are kept in check.

For most of your meals, the spotlight should be on the fatty foods. However, keep in mind that some high-fat foods can also contain high amounts of carbs. And no matter the diet, trans fat in processed foods should always be avoided.

Overall

To succeed with the keto diet, ensure that carbohydrates make up about 5% of your daily caloric intake while protein consists of 15-20% and fat consists of 75-80%. No matter your body weight or height, this ratio applies to all ketogenic dieters.

Types of Ketogenic Diets

The Standard Keto Diet

When keto is practiced in its standard form, the rules apply everyday with no modifications made whatsoever. For seven days a week, the standard keto dieter adheres to a high-fat, moderate-protein, and low-carb diet.

This plan is ideal for those who want to lose weight quickly and is suitable for most people including those who engage in low-intensity exercise such as yoga.

Cyclical Keto Diet

Cyclical keto dieters follow the standard ketogenic diet for 5-6 days a week and consume carbohydrate-rich foods on the remaining days. The objective is to be in ketosis for most of the week and then to temporarily cycle out of ketosis in order to refuel muscle glycogen levels.

To re-enter ketosis after a temporary break, dieters must adhere to a very strict carb limit and perform intermittent fasting on the first day after their high-carb periods.

This type of keto diet is ideal for athletes and bodybuilders who frequently engage in high-intensity exercise and aim to build more muscle. It may also be a suitable option for dieters that have a difficult time resisting cravings.

Targeted Keto Diet

This variation of keto requires you to follow all the same rules of the standard diet except for right before you exercise. 45 minutes to an hour before intense workout sessions, the targeted keto dieter will consume no more than 25-40 grams of carbohydrates (depending on the intensity of their workout) in order to keep their energy levels high.

To be successful with this form of Keto, it's crucial that dieters do not overload on carbohydrates. Too much and your body will not burn enough carbs during exercise to resume ketosis right after.

Targeted keto can be considered a lite version of Cyclical Keto and it's ideal for those who engage in medium to high intensity workouts every week. However, it should be noted that weight loss occurs at a slower rate for the targeted keto dieter.

Mediterranean Keto Diet

If you're more health conscious than most, consider the keto diet with a Mediterranean twist. This variation of the diet emphasises high-quality fats through the consumption of Mediterranean favourites like olive oil and fatty fish while foods like cheese and eggs are eaten in moderation. All processed foods are avoided on this strain of keto.

The Mediterranean keto diet is perfect for dieters who want to significantly lower their cholesterol levels and see greater heart-health benefits overall. The risks with this plan are minimal and in fact, it may be one of the best forms of keto for long-term dieting and general health.

Vegan Keto Diet

Animal products tend to be a staple of the keto diet, but they don't have to be. If you prefer a plant-based approach to keto, then the vegan keto diet may be for you. Instead of eggs, cheese, and meat, a vegan keto diet places more emphasis on plant-based fats like avocado, coconut, and seeds.

While this is certainly a more difficult form of keto, it provides even greater weight loss and heart health benefits for those who are willing to give it a go. This type of keto is ideal for people who already practice a vegan or plant-based lifestyle.

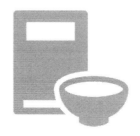

Succeeding with the Keto Diet

Habits to Help You Succeed

Only Keep Keto-Friendly Food

Help yourself resist temptation by removing all non-keto foods from your home. Clear out sugary snacks, whole grains, and starchy vegetables from your fridge. If they aren't easy to access, you'll be far more likely to resist them.

Keep Keto Snacks at the Ready

When cravings hit, give yourself an easier time by having keto-friendly snacks nearby. Make some keto favourites in advance and maintain your supply of easy-to-snack-on goods like cheddar cheese and cucumber sticks.

Drink Lots of Water

A natural appetite suppressant, water will keep you satiated for longer stretches of time. Stay hydrated, and before you snack, consider that maybe your body needs water and not extra calories at this time.

Track Your Intake of Macronutrients

Stay diligent about monitoring your intake of fat, protein, and net carbohydrates. This is the backbone of the keto diet. Get accustomed to reading a nutrition label and looking up nutrition details on your smartphone when eating out.

Plan Your Meals in Advance

Planning your meals in advance will ensure that you don't spend every mealtime counting macros on an empty stomach and giving into temptation because it's easier. Use the recipes in this book to construct a meal plan that works for your time schedule, personal preferences, and keeps you under your daily carb limit.

Connect with others on the Keto Diet

One of the most difficult parts of keto is being around people who get to eat *everything* that you are trying to limit. Whether it's on a dieting app or in real life, connect with people who are also on the same eating plan. This is a proven method for staying disciplined with eating habits. By encouraging each other and sharing your favourite keto-friendly foods, keto dieters are far more likely to resist straying.

Foods to Avoid & Keto-Friendly Substitutes

Cow's Milk & Low-Fat Dairy

Dairy products such as cheese and butter are perfect for the keto diet, but cow's milk and low-fat dairy should be pushed aside. Cow's milk is relatively high in carbs, so replace this with an unsweetened plant-based substitute. If you'd like to eat yoghurt on your diet, avoid flavoured yoghurts and opt for a high-fat, sugar-free alternative.

Instead: plain Greek yoghurt, almond milk, soy milk, and coconut milk for its high fat content.

Starchy Vegetables

We're always taught to eat our greens, but on the keto diet, not all vegetables have a place on your plate. Avoid starchy vegetables such as corn, peas, lentils, artichokes, yams, and potatoes. Keep in mind that anything that grows beneath the ground tends to be high in carbohydrates.

Instead: spinach, asparagus, broccoli, cauliflower, cabbage, courgettes, aubergines, lettuce, kale, and mushrooms.

All Grains

Oats, bread, rice, and pasta should be avoided completely on the keto diet. Just a tiny portion of these high-carb foods can knock you out of ketosis. Thankfully, there are many keto-friendly replacements that work just as well.

Instead: courgetti (pasta made from courgettes), cauliflower bread, cauliflower rice, and broccoli rice.

Sugar

Sugar is a carbohydrate which means it isn't keto-friendly. However, this doesn't mean you have to give up sweet treats entirely. While honey, maple syrup, and refined sugars are an absolute no-go on keto, there are many sugar-free and low-carb sweeteners to satisfy your sweet tooth.

Instead: erythritol, stevia, xylitol, and monk fruit extract.

Most Fruit

The sugars in fruit may be natural but they're sugars all the same. Skip sugary, high-carb fruit such as grapes, bananas, pears, and apples unless you're having a very small amount. Replace these with low-carb fruit, though keep in mind these should also be consumed in moderation.

Instead: avocados, tomatoes, raspberries, strawberries, lemons, and watermelon.

Sugary Condiments

Say no to store-bought ketchup, barbecue sauce, and jam. If you can't do without the ketchup or barbecue sauce, seek out an unsweetened and keto-friendly product. These can be purchased from UK brands such as Hunter Gather or Skinny Food Co.

Instead: sugar-free ketchup, tabasco, mayonnaise, vinaigrette, soy sauce, and butter.

Large Amounts of Nuts or Seeds

Pistachios and cashew nuts should be avoided, with just 100g taking up nearly half of your daily carb allowance – but some nuts and seeds make great additions to the keto diet. Eat nuts and seeds in moderation, ideally no more than 100g per day.

Instead: chia seeds, flaxseeds, sesame seeds, hemp seeds, brazil nuts, and walnuts.

Legumes

Legumes tend to be high in carbohydrates so they are best left aside on the keto diet. Keep kidney beans, pinto beans, black beans, lima beans, and baked beans far away from your plate.

Instead: green beans and black soybeans in moderation.

Beer & Milk or Juice-Based Cocktails

All alcohol will slow weight loss, but if it's a special occasion, you don't have to say no to an alcoholic drink – it just depends on what it is. Say no to beer or any cocktail with a milk or juice base such as a Cosmopolitan or White Russian, but feel free to take a shot of pure spirit.

Instead: dry martini, brandy, whiskey, and one serving of white or red wine.

Recipes

Breakfast

Mediterranean Breakfast Spread

Makes 2 servings
Prep time: 10 minutes | Total: 10 minutes

NET CARBS: 3.6G | PROTEIN: 34G | FIBRE: 3.4G | FAT: 49G
KCAL: 551

INGREDIENTS

- 220g burrata cheese*
- 100g smoked salmon
- 60g assorted olives
- 30g walnuts
- 1 small cucumber
- 1 tomato
- 1 tbsp extra virgin olive oil
- 1 tsp dried oregano or basil

INSTRUCTIONS

1. Chop the tomato into half-slices and the cucumber into thin pieces of your desired width and length.
2. Arrange the chopped vegetables on a chopping board with the burrata cheese, smoked salmon pieces, walnuts, and a small dipping bowl with the assorted olives.
3. Drizzle the entire board with olive oil. Season with salt and pepper.
4. Top everything with a light layer of oregano or basil and serve.

---

*Can be substituted with feta cheese.

Tuna-Stuffed Avocado

Serves 4

Prep time: 15 minutes | Total: 15 minutes

NET CARBS: 2.8G | PROTEIN: 11.4G | FIBRE: 6.9G | FAT: 25G
KCAL: 302

INGREDIENTS

- 140g canned tuna
- 30g mayonnaise
- 2 avocados

- 1 tbsp chopped red onion
- 1 tbsp chopped chives or parsley
- 1 tsp dijon mustard

INSTRUCTIONS

1. Slice the avocado lengthwise and remove the pit. Scoop only half of the green flesh out of each avocado, leaving about 0.5-1cm along each side of the skin.
2. Mash the avocado flesh in a bowl.
3. Add the tuna, mayonnaise, chopped onion, and mustard to the bowl. Stir to combine all ingredients with the avocado flesh.
4. Transfer the mixture into the avocado halves.
5. Serve with a topping of chopped chives or parsley.

Breakfast Egg Bombs

Makes 3 servings (2 per person)
Prep time: 15 minutes | Total: 15 minutes

NET CARBS: 1.8G | PROTEIN: 18.9G | FIBRE: 0.1G | FAT: 34G
KCAL: 390

INGREDIENTS

- 4 hard-boiled eggs
- 3 slices bacon (pre-cooked)
- 180g full-fat cream cheese
- 1 tbsp chopped spring onion
- 1 tbsp chopped chives

INSTRUCTIONS

1. In a bowl, mix together the hard-boiled eggs, cream cheese, spring onion, and chives.
2. Roll the mixture into 9 evenly-sized balls.
3. Place onto a plate and set inside the freezer for 7-10 minutes.
4. While the egg and cream cheese balls are setting, chop the pre-cooked bacon into very small pieces.
5. Roll the egg and cream cheese balls into the bacon bits until coated.
6. Serve or store for later and enjoy.

Almond Flour Waffles

Serves 2

Prep time: 10 minutes | Cook time: 20 minutes | Total: 30 minutes

NET CARBS: 2.6G | PROTEIN: 8.7G | FIBRE: 1.6G | FAT: 46G
KCAL: 474

INGREDIENTS

- 100g blanched almond flour
- 60ml heavy cream
- 2 eggs
- 1 tsp vanilla extract
- 2 tbsp erythritol
- 2 tbsp coconut oil
- 2 tbsp butter
- 1 tsp baking powder

INSTRUCTIONS

1. Preheat your waffle maker and lightly grease with coconut oil.
2. In a bowl, beat the eggs and whisk with vanilla extract, heavy cream, and erythritol.
3. Slowly incorporate almond flour and baking powder into the mixture.
4. Add a pinch of salt and stir until completely smooth.
5. Spoon the waffle batter into the pre-heated waffle maker.
6. Cook for about 5 minutes or until waffles are golden.
7. Continue with the rest of the waffle batter until finished.
8. Serve with a tablespoon of butter for every two waffles.

Keto Smoothie Bowl

Makes 1 serving
Prep time: 5 minutes | Total: 5 minutes

NET CARBS: 9G | PROTEIN: 5G | FIBRE: 12G | FAT: 41.4G
KCAL: 445

INGREDIENTS

- 100ml unsweetened almond milk
- 80ml coconut milk
- 80g frozen strawberries or raspberries (unsweetened)

- ½ avocado
- 3 drops of stevia
- 1 tsp coconut flakes (optional)
- ½ tsp chia seeds (optional)

INSTRUCTIONS

1. Add the almond milk, coconut milk, fruit, and stevia to a high-speed blender and blend until smooth.
2. Pour into a bowl.
3. Serve with a topping of coconut flakes and chia seeds, and enjoy.

Spanish Baked Eggs

Makes 4 servings

Prep time: 15 minutes | Cook time: 20 minutes | Total: 35 minutes

NET CARBS: 4.4G | PROTEIN: 25.4G | FIBRE: 2.9G | FAT: 32.8G
KCAL: 442

INGREDIENTS

- 400g chopped tomatoes (1 can)
- 225g chorizo
- 4 eggs
- 2 garlic cloves
- 1 red bell pepper
- 1 onion
- 1 lime
- 1 tsp paprika
- ½ tsp cumin
- 55g grated parmesan cheese
- 1 tbsp extra virgin olive oil
- 2 tsps chopped parsley or cilantro (optional)

INSTRUCTIONS

1. Preheat the oven to 200°C / 180°C (fan).
2. Dice the chorizo, bell peppers, and onion. Mince the garlic.
3. Heat an ovenproof pan with olive oil over medium heat. If you don't own an ovenproof pan, use any frying pan, but you'll need to transfer the sauce into an oven-safe dish later on.
4. Cook the diced chorizo and onion until the meat is lightly browned, about 4 minutes.
5. Add the minced garlic and bell peppers. Cook for 1 more minute or until the garlic is fragrant.

6. Pour in the canned tomatoes. Squeeze all the juice out of the lime into your sauce. Season with salt, pepper, paprika, and cumin.

7. Let the sauce simmer for 4-5 more minutes or until it has thickened. If you're not using an ovenproof pan, transfer the sauce to an oven-safe dish once it has finished thickening.

8. Off heat, make four holes or wells in the tomato sauce with a spoon.

9. Crack an egg into each hole, then top with grated parmesan cheese.

10. Bake for 7-10 minutes, depending on your egg consistency preference.

11. Serve with chopped parsley or cilantro.

Keto Croque Madame

Makes 2 servings

Prep time: 15 minutes | Cook time: 30 minutes | Total: 45 minutes

NET CARBS: 3.3G | PROTEIN: 59.3 | FIBRE: 1.4G | FAT: 57.1G
KCAL: 783

INGREDIENTS

For the keto bread:

♦ 120g grated cheddar cheese

♦ 3 large eggs

♦ ½ tsp garlic powder

♦ ½ tsp Italian seasoning

For the filling and topping:

♦ 15g grated parmesan or cheddar cheese

♦ 4 slices of gruyere or swiss cheese

♦ 4 slices of ham

♦ 2 large eggs

♦ ½ red onion

INSTRUCTIONS

1. Preheat the oven to 180°C / 160°C (fan).
2. Begin making the keto bread by beating the eggs in a bowl and mixing with the grated cheddar cheese. Add the Italian seasoning and garlic powder.
3. Pour the keto bread batter into a baking pan covered in parchment paper. Make sure it's in an even layer. Bake for 20 minutes.
4. Meanwhile, dice the red onion to prepare for your filling.
5. Remove the keto bread from the oven and let it cool.
6. Increase the heat of the oven to 220°C / 200°C (fan).

7. Cut out four evenly-sized pieces of keto bread to make two sandwiches. Divide accordingly.

8. On each sandwich, layer one slice of ham followed by one slice of cheese, then repeat. Add the diced onion then close the sandwich.

9. Bake for 8-10 minutes.

10. Meanwhile, cook two fried eggs.

11. Remove the two sandwiches from the oven. Top with grated parmesan or cheddar cheese and one fried egg for each sandwich.

12. Serve your keto croque madames and enjoy.

Feta & Mushroom Egg Muffins

Makes 4 servings (2 muffins per person)
Prep time: 10 minutes | Cook time: 20 minutes | Total: 30 minutes

NET CARBS: 1G | PROTEIN: 15.5G | FIBRE: 0.7G | FAT: 12.7G
KCAL: 184

INGREDIENTS

- 8 large eggs
- 50g feta cheese crumbles
- 50g mushrooms
- 30g red or yellow bell peppers
- 3 garlic cloves
- 1 tbsp chopped onion
- 1 tsp basil (optional)

INSTRUCTIONS

1. Preheat the oven to 180°C / 160°C (fan).
2. Dice the garlic and bell peppers. Slice the mushrooms.
3. Generously spray a muffin tin with cooking spray.
4. In a bowl, whisk the eggs with salt and pepper. Combine with the chopped garlic and onion, then pour into each cup of the muffin tin until about halfway.
5. Top the egg mixture with sliced mushrooms, bell peppers, and feta cheese crumbles.
6. Bake for 14-16 minutes.
7. Serve with basil sprinkled on top.

Herb & Prawn Omelette

Makes 4 servings
Prep time: 5 minutes | Cook time: 10 minutes | Total: 15 minutes

NET CARBS: 3G | PROTEIN: 22.8G | FIBRE: 0.5G | FAT: 23G
KCAL: 310

INGREDIENTS

- 160g chopped prawns (pre-cooked)
- 100ml heavy whipping cream
- 8 large eggs
- 1 spring onion
- 4 tbsps chives
- 2 tbsps parsley
- 2 tbsps dill
- 1 tbsp butter

INSTRUCTIONS

1. Finely slice the spring onion.
2. In a medium bowl, whisk together the eggs, heavy whipping cream, salt, and herbs.
3. Heat a skillet with butter at medium-high heat.
4. Pour the egg mixture into the pan and allow to set.
5. As the edges begin to set, use your spatula or wooden spoon to pull the egg over.
6. Add the prawns to the pan. Season with salt and pepper.
7. Cook until the prawns are hot and the egg has fully set.
8. Top with spring onions and serve.

Lunch

One-Pan Garlic Chicken & Broccoli

Makes 2 servings

Prep time: 10 minutes | Cook time: 25 minutes | Total: 35 minutes

NET CARBS: 7.5G | PROTEIN: 17.3G | FIBRE: 3.9G | FAT: 34.3G
KCAL: 415

INGREDIENTS

- 200g broccoli florets
- 120g boneless chicken thighs
- 150g cherry tomatoes
- 60g cream cheese
- 5 garlic cloves
- 2 tbsps extra virgin olive oil
- ½ tsp of Italian seasoning

INSTRUCTIONS

1. Mince the garlic and halve the cherry tomatoes.
2. Heat the olive oil in a large skillet or pan at medium-high heat. Add the chicken thighs. Season with salt and pepper. Cook until golden for about 4-5 minutes on each side.
3. Add minced garlic to the pan and cook with the chicken thighs for 1 minute.
4. Add broccoli, tomatoes, and cream cheese to the pan. Cook with Italian seasoning for 4 minutes or until broccoli is tender and cooked through.
5. Serve and enjoy.

Caprese Stuffed Mushrooms

Makes 2 servings

Prep time: 10 minutes | Cook time: 25 minutes | Total: 35 minutes

NET CARBS: 4.7G | PROTEIN: 26.9G | FIBRE: 3.3G | FAT: 32G
KCAL: 425

INGREDIENTS

- 4 portobello mushrooms
- 3 garlic clove
- 120g baby tomatoes
- 2 tbsps extra virgin olive oil
- 4 mozzarella balls
- 2 tsps fresh or dried basil
- ½ tsp balsamic vinegar

INSTRUCTIONS

1. Preheat the oven to 200°C / 180°C (fan).
2. Chop the baby tomatoes in half and dice the garlic. Pat-dry the mozzarella balls and thinly slice them.
3. Twist off stems from the mushrooms and scoop out the gills from under the mushroom cap.
4. In a small bowl, coat the mushrooms in olive oil and salt to taste.
5. Bake mushrooms for 9-10 minutes or until mushrooms have softened.
6. In the same oiled bowl, combine the mozzarella cheese, chopped tomatoes, diced garlic, and half of the basil. Season with salt and pepper. Mix well.
7. Remove the portobello mushrooms from the oven. Fill with the Caprese mixture.
8. Bake stuffed mushrooms for 11-14 minutes or until tomatoes have softened.

9. Add a dash of balsamic vinegar to each mushroom.

10. Top with any remaining basil and serve.

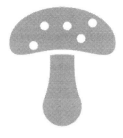

Watermelon & Prosciutto Salad

Makes 2 servings
Prep time: 15 minutes | Total: 15 minutes

NET CARBS: 4.9G | PROTEIN: 26.5G | FIBRE: 5.8G | FAT: 41.5G
KCAL: 561

INGREDIENTS

- 280g rocket or spinach
- 180g diced watermelon
- 120g crumbled feta cheese
- 8 slices of prosciutto
- 2 red onions

- 3 tbsps extra virgin olive oil
- 2 tbsps balsamic or white vinegar
- 1 tbsp mustard
- 1 tsp salt
- 1 bunch fresh mint (optional)

INSTRUCTIONS

1. Dice the red onions. Set aside while you make the dressing.
2. In a bowl, combine the olive oil, vinegar, mustard, and salt. Stir or whisk together.
3. Add the rocket, shredded prosciutto, and onions to the bowl. Toss until the leaves are fully coated in dressing.
4. Once mixed, add the diced tomato and crumbled feta cheese on top. Lightly toss, but not too much or the salad will get soggy.
5. Serve with fresh mint leaves and enjoy.

Courgette Grilled Cheese

Makes 4 servings
Prep time: 15 minutes | Cook time: 20 minutes | Total: 35 minutes

NET CARBS: 1.6G | PROTEIN: 14.7G | FIBRE: 1.7G | FAT: 20G
KCAL: 255

INGREDIENTS

- 150g grated cheddar or gruyere cheese
- 20g grated parmesan cheese
- 30g almond flour
- 2 courgettes
- 1 egg
- 1 spring onion
- 1 tbsp of butter

INSTRUCTIONS

1. Grate the courgettes with a box grater or food processor. Chop the spring onions finely.
2. Use a kitchen towel to remove any excess moisture. Press firmly against the courgette to ensure it's as dry as possible, then put away the wet kitchen towel.
3. In a bowl, combine the grated courgette with the spring onions, almond flour, parmesan cheese, and egg. Season with salt and pepper.
4. Heat up a pan with butter at medium-high heat.
5. Spoon three tablespoons of your courgette mixture onto the pan. Using your spatula, shape into a rectangle or square so it looks roughly bread-shaped.
6. Cook about 4-5 minutes on each side or until golden.

7. Remove the finished courgette 'toast' and repeat step 5 until all of your courgette mixture is gone.

8. Reduce the heat on your pan to medium.

9. Place one of your finished courgette toasts back on the pan. Top with your chosen grated cheese until fully covered. Place another courgette toast on top to create a sandwich.

10. Cook for about 1-2 minutes or until the cheese has melted to your liking.

11. Serve and enjoy.

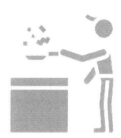

Chicken Butterhead Lettuce Wraps

Makes 4 servings

Prep time: 15 minutes | Cook time: 10 minutes | Total: 25 minutes

NET CARBS: 2.5G | PROTEIN: 21.5G | FIBRE: 3.8G | FAT: 30.3G
KCAL: 385

INGREDIENTS

For the wraps:

♦ 450g boneless chicken thighs

♦ 3 garlic cloves

♦ 1 spring onion

♦ 1 avocado

♦ 2 tsps ground ginger

♦ 4 butter lettuce heads

♦ 1 tbsp extra virgin olive oil

For the dipping sauce:

♦ 2 tsps rice wine vinegar

♦ 1 tsp Blue Dragon Fish Sauce

♦ ½ tsp freshly squeezed lime juice

INSTRUCTIONS

1. Dice the garlic, spring onion, and avocado. Set aside.
2. Careful to not touch your raw ingredients, dice the boneless chicken thighs into small bite-sized pieces.
3. Add olive oil to a pan over medium-high heat. Cook the diced chicken thighs until it is no longer pink, about 7-8 minutes.
4. Add the garlic, spring onion, and ground ginger to the pan. Season with salt and pepper. Cook together until fragrant, about 1-2 minutes.
5. Pull apart the butterhead lettuce so you have separate cups of lettuce.

6. Assemble the wraps by spooning the cooked chicken mixture into each lettuce cup. Top with diced avocado.

7. In a small bowl, combine the rice wine vinegar, fish sauce, and lime juice.

8. Serve the lettuce wraps with dipping sauce.

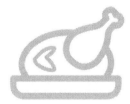

Salmon Sushi Rolls

Makes 2 servings
Prep time: 25 minutes | Total: 25 minutes

NET CARBS: 1G | PROTEIN: 14G | FIBRE: 8.6G | FAT: 26.8G
KCAL: 340

INGREDIENTS

- 4 sheets of roasted seaweed (nori)
- 100g smoked salmon
- 100g full-fat cream cheese
- 1 avocado
- ½ cucumber
- 2 tbsps soy sauce (optional)

INSTRUCTIONS

1. Place the sheet of roasted seaweed on a dry chopping board. With a sharp knife, cut each sheet of nori into 4 pieces. Repeat with the rest of the seaweed until you have 16 squares of nori.
2. Cut the cucumber into thin slices. Chop the avocado and smoked salmon into 16 pieces of a similar length to the cucumber, but thicker in width.
3. Fill a small bowl with water and set it down next to the chopping board.
4. Scoop a heaping teaspoon of cream cheese onto the nori sheet. Arrange lengthways with your fingers.
5. Add a piece of smoked salmon and avocado lengthways to the seaweed sheet, followed by a couple of pieces of cucumber.

6. Dip your fingertips into the bowl of water, then carefully seal up the sushi roll. The water should make it easier to close the seams.

7. Repeat until all the sushi rolls have been made.

8. Serve alone or with soy sauce.

Garlic Butter Prawns

Makes 4 servings
Prep time: 5 minutes | Cook time: 20 minutes | Total: 25 minutes

NET CARBS: 5.6G | PROTEIN: 31.9G | FIBRE: 1.2G | FAT: 29.6G
KCAL: 425

INGREDIENTS

- 450g prawns
- 200ml heavy whipping cream
- 90g spinach
- 50g grated parmesan cheese
- 5 garlic cloves
- 1 onion
- 2 tbsps butter
- 1 tsp Italian seasoning

INSTRUCTIONS

1. Finely dice the onion and garlic.
2. Heat a pan with butter over medium-high heat. Add the prawns and cook for 2 minutes on each side. Before flipping, add the garlic to the pan. Set aside when the prawns are pink.
3. Add the chopped onions to the pan and fry until translucent for about 3-4 minutes.
4. Reduce the heat to medium-low and pour in the heavy whipping cream. Season well with salt and pepper.
5. Add the spinach and parmesan cheese to the simmering cream sauce. Mix cheese into the sauce. Simmer and stir for 3-5 minutes or until thickened.
6. Return the prawns and garlic to the pan. Add the Italian seasoning and stir to fully coat the prawns in sauce and herbs.
7. Serve and enjoy.

Club Salad

Makes 2 servings
Prep time: 10 minutes | Total: 10 minutes

NET CARBS: 6.3G | PROTEIN: 21.3G | FIBRE: 2G | FAT: 28.9G
KCAL: 392

INGREDIENTS

- 300g chopped Romaine lettuce
- 150g cucumber
- 110g cheddar or Edam cheese
- 15g cherry tomatoes
- 2 hard-boiled eggs
- ½ red onion
- 2 tbsps sour cream
- 1 tbsp mayonnaise
- 1 tsp heavy whipping cream

INSTRUCTIONS

1. Dice the red onion, halve the cherry tomatoes, and quarter-slice the cucumber into bite-sized pieces.
2. Slice the hard-boiled eggs into wedges and cube your chosen cheese.
3. In a separate bowl, combine the mayonnaise, sour cream, and heavy whipping cream. Stir to fully combine and make a dressing.
4. Add lettuce to a serving bowl along with the onion, cucumber, tomatoes, and cheese cubes. Scoop the dressing onto the greens and mix well.
5. Top with the wedges of hard-boiled egg and serve.

Cheesy Spinach & Tomato Pie

Makes 4 servings

Prep time: 5 minutes | Cook time: 35 minutes | Total: 40 minutes

NET CARBS: 1.5G | PROTEIN: 22.5G | FIBRE: 2.7G | FAT: 22.6G
KCAL: 317

INGREDIENTS

- 300g spinach
- 160g shredded cheddar cheese
- 50g crumbled feta cheese
- 5 large eggs

- 2 tomatoes
- ½ onion
- 1 tsp basil

INSTRUCTIONS

1. Preheat the oven to 200°C / 180°C (fan).
2. Slice the tomatoes and dice the half onion.
3. In a bowl, whisk the eggs.
4. Once smooth, add the diced onion, shredded cheddar, crumbled feta, and spinach. Season with salt and pepper. Stir to combine with the eggs.
5. Pour the egg, spinach, and cheese mixture into a greased baking pan.
6. Bake for 30 minutes, taking the pie out after the 15-minute mark to top with a single layer of tomato slices before continuing to cook. Remove from the oven once the edges begin to brown.
7. Serve with a topping of basil.

Dinner

Lemon Cream Salmon

Makes 2 servings
Prep time: 5 minutes | Cook time: 10 minutes | Total: 15 minutes

NET CARBS: 5.3G | PROTEIN: 36.7G | FIBRE: 0.4G | FAT: 45.9G
KCAL: 570

INGREDIENTS

- 150ml heavy whipping cream
- 2 salmon fillets
- 2 garlic cloves
- 1 shallot
- 1 tbsp lemon juice
- 1 tbsp extra virgin olive oil or coconut oil
- 1 tbsp parsley (optional)
- 2 lemon wedges (optional)

INSTRUCTIONS

1. Mince the garlic and finely slice the shallot.
2. Heat olive oil in a pan over medium-high heat.
3. Cook salmon until lightly browned on both sides, then remove from the pan.
4. Reduce heat to medium. Add the garlic and chopped shallots. Cook for 1 minute or until fragrant.
5. Add the heavy whipping cream to the pan. Bring to a simmer and stir occasionally. Cook until thickened, about 4-5 minutes.
6. Add lemon juice to the cream sauce. Season with salt and pepper.
7. Place cooked salmon into the sauce to heat up for about 2-3 minutes.
8. Top with parsley and serve with lemon wedges on the side.

Pork Loin with Cauliflower Mash

Makes 2 servings

Prep time: 25 minutes | Cook time: 35 minutes | Total: 1 hour

NET CARBS: 2.1G | PROTEIN: 68G | FIBRE: 7.3G | FAT: 21.8G
KCAL: 530

INGREDIENTS

- 475g pork tenderloin
- 1 medium cauliflower head (575g)
- 1 tbsp extra virgin olive oil
- 2 garlic cloves
- 1 tbsp butter
- ½ tsp Italian seasoning

INSTRUCTIONS

1. Preheat the oven to 200°C / 180°C (fan).
2. Mince the garlic.
3. In a bowl, combine the olive oil, minced garlic, Italian seasoning, salt, and pepper.
4. Rub or brush each pork loin with the olive oil and garlic mixture.
5. Sear your pork loins in a pan over medium-high heat, about 3 minutes on each side.
6. After searing, place your pork loin in the oven and roast for 12-15 minutes, depending on the thickness of your pork.
7. Boil a pot of water.
8. While water heats, cut the cauliflower into small florets.
9. Add cauliflower to boiling water and cook until tender for about 6-8 minutes.

10. Drain water and keep cauliflower in the warm pot. Add butter. Season with salt and pepper to taste.

11. Mash the buttered cauliflower with a hand-held masher or a blender. Continue until no lumps remain.

12. Remove pork from the oven once its internal temperature has reached 63°C.

13. Serve together and enjoy.

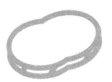

Eggplant Parmigiana

Makes 4 servings

Prep time: 15 minutes | Cook time: 50 minutes | Total: 1 hour 5 minutes

NET CARBS: 2.5G | PROTEIN: 35.2G | FIBRE: 22.4G | FAT: 32.2G
KCAL: 590

INGREDIENTS

- 800g chopped tomatoes (2 cans)
- 250g ricotta cheese
- 200g shredded cheddar cheese
- 100g grated parmesan cheese
- 4 medium aubergines

- 3 garlic cloves
- 1 onion
- 1 bay leaf
- 1 tbsp extra virgin olive oil
- 1 tsp Italian seasoning

INSTRUCTIONS

1. Preheat the oven to 200°C / 180°C (fan).
2. Finely dice the onion and garlic. Slice the aubergines lengthways into pieces of about 1cm thickness.
3. Arrange the aubergine slices on a baking tray. Rub with olive oil. Season with salt and pepper. Bake for 20 minutes, turning them over halfway through.
4. Meanwhile, heat a pan with olive oil over medium heat. Add the onion and cook for 3-4 minutes until lightly golden.
5. Add the garlic and cook for 1 more minute until fragrant.
6. Pour the chopped tomatoes into the pan. Add the bay leaf and Italian seasoning, then stir to combine flavours. Season well with salt and pepper.

7. Cover and bring to a simmer. Let the sauce sit and thicken until you're ready to use it. Ideally, it should simmer for at least 20 minutes.*

8. While the sauce thickens, remove the cooked aubergine slices from the oven. Dab gently with a kitchen towel to reduce oiliness.

9. In a bowl, combine the ricotta and shredded cheddar cheese.

10. Spoon an even layer of the thickened tomato sauce onto the bottom of an oven-safe casserole dish.

11. Follow with a layer of aubergine slices.

12. Spoon the cheese blend on top of the aubergine slices.

13. Repeat steps 10-13 until the sauce, cheese mixture, and eggplant slices are finished.

14. Top with grated parmesan cheese.

15. Cover with aluminium foil and bake for another 20-25 minutes.

16. Serve and enjoy.

*For a very thick sauce, cook before the aubergines and allow to simmer for up to 1 hour.

Chicken Rogan Josh

Makes 4 servings

Prep time: 15 minutes | Cook time: 45 minutes | Total: 1 hour

NET CARBS: 9.7G | PROTEIN: 34G | FIBRE: 5.3G | FAT: 10.3G
KCAL: 295

INGREDIENTS

- 420g chicken thighs
- 400g chopped tomatoes (1 can)
- 2 tomatoes
- 4 garlic cloves
- 2 onions
- 1 chicken stock cube
- 2 tbsps curry powder
- 2 tsps ground turmeric
- 2 tsps ground coriander
- 2 tsps chili powder*
- ½ tsp ground cardamom
- 150g plain, full-fat Greek yoghurt
- 1 tsp extra virgin olive oil

INSTRUCTIONS

1. Preheat the oven to 200°C / 180°C (fan).
2. Boil a kettle with water.
3. Chop the onions and tomatoes into wedges. Crush the garlic cloves.
4. On a separate chopping board, remove the bones from the chicken thighs and dice into bite-sized pieces.
5. Heat an oven-proof pot with olive oil at medium-high heat.
6. Add the onions, tomatoes, and garlic to the pot. Season with salt.
7. Add the curry powder, turmeric, coriander, chili powder, and ground cardamom. Stir into the mixture.

---

*In the case of sensitivity to spice, use only ½ teaspoon of chili powder.

8. Pour in 100ml of hot water and all of the chopped tomatoes. Stir in the chicken stock cube.

9. Add the diced chicken thighs to the pot.

10. Once boiling, remove the pot from the stove and place into the oven. Bake for 35 minutes until the chicken is fully cooked.

11. Serve with a side of plain yoghurt.

Garlic & Mushroom Steak Bites

Makes 2 servings
Prep time: 10 minutes | Cook time: 10 minutes | Total: 20 minutes

NET CARBS: 2.5G | PROTEIN: 54.3G | FIBRE: 2.2G | FAT: 29G
KCAL: 504

INGREDIENTS

- 450g rump or sirloin steak
- 170g mushrooms
- 1 courgette
- 3 garlic cloves

- 2 tbsps butter
- 1 tbsp extra virgin olive oil
- ½ tsp thyme
- ½ tsp rosemary

INSTRUCTIONS

1. Quarter-slice the courgette into pieces about 1-2cm thick. Mince the garlic and chop the mushrooms to your desired thickness.
2. Slice the steak into bite-sized pieces of 2-3cm thick.
3. Heat olive oil in a pan at medium-high heat. Add the steak bites. Season with salt and pepper. Cook for about 2-3 minutes or until steak bites have begun to brown.
4. Add the sliced mushrooms, courgette pieces, garlic, thyme, rosemary, and butter to the pan.
5. Cover and cook for 4-6 minutes until the courgettes are tender.
6. Serve and enjoy.

Lamb, Tomato & Coconut Curry

Makes 4 servings

Prep time: 5 minutes | Cook time: 20 minutes | Total: 25 minutes

> NET CARBS:4.1G | PROTEIN: 42.4G | FIBRE: 4.6G | FAT: 29.2G
> KCAL: 483

INGREDIENTS

- 550g diced lamb
- 120g spinach
- 200g chopped tomatoes (½ can)
- 250ml coconut cream
- 1 lime
- 2 onion
- 2 garlic cloves
- 2 tsps ground ginger
- 1 tsp coriander
- ½ tsp turmeric
- ½ tsp cumin
- ½ tsp paprika
- 1 tbsp extra virgin olive oil or coconut oil

INSTRUCTIONS

1. Mince the garlic and finely chop the onions.
2. Heat a pot with olive or coconut oil at high heat.
3. Cook the diced lamb for 3 minutes, stirring occasionally.
4. Add the diced onions and garlic. Cook for 1-2 minutes.
5. When the onions begin to soften, add the ground ginger, coriander, turmeric, cumin, and paprika to the pan.
6. Stir for 30 seconds to combine and release the flavours of the spices.
7. Pour in the chopped tomatoes and coconut cream. Add the spinach and stir well to fully combine all ingredients.

8. Reduce the heat to medium-low and cover. Let it simmer for 8-10 minutes until the sauce looks like it has thickened and the spinach has softened.
9. Season with salt and pepper. Squeeze the juice from a lime into the pot.
10. Serve alone or with cauliflower rice.

Alfredo Courgetti Noodles

Makes 4 servings
Prep time: 5 minutes | Cook time: 5 minutes | Total: 10 minutes

NET CARBS: 2.4G | PROTEIN: 6.7G | FIBRE: 1.7G | FAT: 17.3G
KCAL: 199

INGREDIENTS

- 600g courgetti noodles
- 120ml heavy whipping cream
- 50g grated parmesan cheese
- 2 garlic cloves
- 1 tbsp butter
- ½ tsp Italian seasoning
- 2 tsps parsley (optional)

INSTRUCTIONS

1. Finely dice the garlic.
2. Heat a pan with butter over medium-high heat.
3. Add the garlic and courgetti noodles to the pan. Cook for 1-2 minutes until the noodles start to soften. Stir occasionally.
4. Pour in the heavy whipping cream.
5. Reduce the heat to low heat and allow to simmer for 2 minutes.
6. Stir in the Italian seasoning and most of the parmesan cheese. Season well with salt and pepper.
7. Top with parsley and serve with the remaining parmesan cheese.

Chicken & Broccoli Casserole

Makes 4 servings

Prep time: 15 minutes | Cook time: 15 minutes | Total: 30 minutes

> NET CARBS: 6.8G | PROTEIN: 35.8G | FIBRE: 3.7G | FAT: 33.2G
> KCAL: 480

INGREDIENTS

- 560g broccoli
- 300g shredded or chopped chicken (pre-cooked)
- 180g cream cheese
- 110ml heavy whipping cream
- 110ml unsweetened almond milk
- 100g shredded cheddar or mozzarella cheese
- 50g grated parmesan cheese
- 2 garlic cloves

INSTRUCTIONS

1. Mince the garlic. Chop the broccoli into bite-sized florets.
2. Bring a pot of water to boil and add the broccoli florets to salted water. Boil for 4-5 minutes then transfer to a mixing bowl.
3. Preheat the broiler.
4. In a pan over low heat, add the cream cheese, unsweetened almond milk, heavy whipping cream, and minced garlic. Season with salt and pepper. Stir to combine.
5. In the mixing bowl, combine the creamy cheese mixture with the chicken and broccoli.
6. Spread the broccoli and cheese blend onto the bottom of an oven-safe casserole dish. Top with grated parmesan cheese.

7. Broil for about 3-5 minutes or until the cheese looks golden. Time will vary depending on the broiler.

8. Serve and enjoy.

Keto Hawaiian Pizza

Makes 2 servings
Prep time: 20 minutes | Cook time: 50 minutes | Total: 1 hour 10 minutes

NET CARBS: 6.3G | PROTEIN: 37.2G | FIBRE: 6.5G | FAT: 20.5G
KCAL: 413

INGREDIENTS

For the pizza crust:

- 280g cauliflower florets
- 100g grated parmesan cheese
- 1 large egg
- ½ tsp onion powder
- ½ tsp extra virgin olive oil

For the pizza topping:

- 120g shredded mozzarella cheese
- 100g tomato paste
- 75g sliced ham or Canadian bacon
- 60g finely diced pineapple
- 1 tsp basil
- 1 tsp oregano
- 1 tsp garlic powder

INSTRUCTIONS

1. Preheat the oven to 200°C / 180°C (fan).
2. Begin by ricing the cauliflower florets. For the most ease, use a food processor. However, a box grater with small holes can also be used though this requires a bit more time and effort.
3. Heat a pan with no oil at medium-high heat. Cook the cauliflower until extremely soft, about 10 minutes. Stir frequently to ensure that all moisture is cooked off.

4. While the cauliflower is cooking, beat the egg in a large bowl. Once smooth, add the parmesan cheese and onion powder.

5. Remove the fried cauliflower from the pan once it looks soft and dry. Mix into the large bowl with the egg and cheese mixture until you have a dough. Make sure to fully combine, using a spatula if necessary.

6. Lightly grease some parchment paper with olive oil and transfer the cauliflower dough. Separate the dough into two balls, but if you have a tray that fits a large-sized pizza, feel free to keep it as one.

7. Flatten the dough with your hands to your desired thickness, but no less than 0.5cm and no more than 1cm. You may use a rolling pin for this step if you prefer. Lastly, raise the edges of the dough to form the pizza crust.

8. Bake for 20 minutes.

9. While the pizza crust bakes, heat a pan over medium-low heat. Add the tomato paste and about 50-60ml of water.

10. Use your spatula to stir and fully blend the paste and water. Simmer for 3-4 minutes or until the sauce looks slightly thickened.

11. Season with salt and pepper. Stir in the basil, oregano, and garlic powder.

12. Allow the un-topped pizza to cool for 3-5 minutes before adding your toppings.

13. Add a layer of tomato sauce to the pizza, followed by another layer of mozzarella cheese. Top with bacon or ham and pineapple chunks.

14. Bake for 10 minutes.

15. Serve and enjoy.

Creamy White Chicken Chili

Makes 4 servings
Prep time: 15 minutes | Cook time: 35 minutes | Total: 50 minutes

> NET CARBS: 3.4G | PROTEIN: 43G | FIBRE: 1.1G | FAT: 34.8G
> KCAL: 519

INGREDIENTS

- 450g boneless chicken breasts
- 140g green chili peppers (1 can)
- 120g full-fat cream cheese
- 400ml chicken broth
- 60ml heavy whipping cream
- 80g shredded cheddar cheese
- 3 garlic cloves
- 1 red bell pepper
- 1 onion
- 1 tbsp butter
- 1 tsp ground cumin

INSTRUCTIONS

1. Dice the onion, garlic, and red pepper. On a separate chopping board, slice the chicken breasts into bite-sized pieces.
2. Heat a large pot with butter on medium-high heat.
3. Add the chicken pieces and onion to the pan. Season with salt and pepper. Cook for 4-5 minutes until the onions begin to look translucent.
4. Add the bell peppers and cook for an additional 4-5 minutes until the chicken looks golden.
5. Stir in the cumin, garlic, chili peppers, and chicken broth.
6. Bring to a boil then reduce the heat to low and allow to simmer for 10 minutes.

7. Put the cream cheese in a bowl and microwave for 20-30 seconds until it's stirrable.

8. Combine with the heavy whipping cream and cheddar cheese.

9. Add the cheese mixture to the simmering pot, making sure to stir quickly so that it blends with the chicken soup and doesn't sink to the bottom.

10. Simmer for another 10 minutes.

11. Top with any extra shredded cheese and enjoy.

Sides & Snacks

Bacon Jalapeno Poppers

Makes 4 servings (2-3 per person)
Prep time: 15 minutes | Cook time: 20 minutes | Total: 35 minutes

> NET CARBS: 2.3G | PROTEIN: 13.1G | FIBRE: 0.6G | FAT: 22.4G
> KCAL: 264

INGREDIENTS

- 5 jalapenos
- 100g full-fat cream cheese
- 20g diced onions
- 50g bacon bits (pre-cooked)
- 100g shredded cheddar cheese
- ½ tsp garlic powder

INSTRUCTIONS

1. Preheat the oven to 190°C / 170°C (fan).
2. Scoop out the seeds from the jalapenos then cut lengthwise.
3. In a bowl, combine the cream cheese, diced onions, and bacon bits. Season with salt, pepper, and garlic powder.
4. Fill each hollowed jalapeno with your cream cheese mixture.
5. Top each stuffed jalapeno with shredded cheddar cheese.
6. Bake for 20 minutes until the cheese has melted and the jalapenos look tender.
7. Serve and enjoy.

Halloumi Fries

Makes 3 servings

Prep time: 5 minutes | Cook time: 10 minutes | Total: 15 minutes

NET CARBS: 0G (0%) | PROTEIN: 18.7G | FIBRE: | FAT: 24G
KCAL: 293

INGREDIENTS

- ◆ 1 pack or 225g halloumi cheese
- ◆ 1 tbsp avocado oil or coconut oil

INSTRUCTIONS

1. Dry the halloumi gently with a kitchen towel. Cut into fries of your desired thickness, but no thinner than 1 cm.
2. Add a dash of your chosen oil to a frying pan at medium-high heat.
3. Use a pair of tongs to place halloumi fries on the pan. Multiple at a time is fine as long as they are not touching. Otherwise, they may stick together.
4. Cook the halloumi until golden, about 2 minutes on each side.
5. Serve alone or with a keto-friendly sauce, such as Hunter & Gather's Unsweetened Smokey Barbecue Sauce or Unsweetened Classic Tomato Ketchup.

Cucumber Shrimp Bites with Guacamole

Makes 2 servings
Prep time: 15 minutes | Cook time: 10 minutes | Total: 25 minutes

NET CARBS: 4G | PROTEIN: 4.5G | FIBRE: 3G | FAT: 9G
KCAL: 113

INGREDIENTS

- 100g large shrimp (deveined and peeled)
- 1 cucumber
- 1 avocado
- ½ lime
- 1 tbsp of extra virgin olive oil or coconut oil
- ¼ tsp cayenne pepper
- ¼ tsp garlic powder

INSTRUCTIONS

1. Cut cucumber so there is one slice for every piece of shrimp.
2. In a bowl, coat shrimp in olive oil, onion powder, cayenne pepper, salt, and black pepper.
3. Cook shrimp over medium-high heat in your chosen oil. About 3 minutes on each side.
4. Mash the avocado in a bowl. Squeeze lime juice and season with salt. Combine into a blended mixture.
5. Spoon avocado mixture so it covers each cucumber slice. Top with shrimp pieces.
6. Serve with lime wedges as a garnish and enjoy.

Teriyaki Eggplant

Makes 2 servings

Prep time: 15 minutes | Cook time: 15 minutes | Total: 30 minutes

NET CARBS: 1.3G | PROTEIN: 5.1G | FIBRE: 10.4G | FAT: 14.8G
KCAL: 221

INGREDIENTS

- 1 medium aubergine (550g)
- 1 spring onion
- 2 garlic cloves
- 55ml soy sauce
- 30ml sesame oil

- 1 tbsp erythritol
- 1 tsp ground ginger
- ½ tsp apple cider vinegar
- ½ tsp sesame seeds

INSTRUCTIONS

1. Mince the garlic and finely slice the spring onion.

2. Prepare the aubergine by removing the stem and slicing it lengthways into pieces about 0.5cm thick.

3. In a bowl, combine the soy sauce, sesame oil, mirin, erythritol, and apple cider vinegar.

4. Fry the garlic, ground ginger, and sesame seeds in a pan on medium-low heat for 30-45 seconds until fragrant.

5. Off heat, combine the sauce blend with the cooked spices and sesame seeds.

6. Coat the eggplant slices in the teriyaki sauce, using a brush or carefully with a spoon. They should be fully coated but not drenched. If there is sauce left over, save this in a small bowl and use it later as a dipping sauce.

7. Once each slice is coated in teriyaki, cook in a pan on medium-high heat for about 2-3 minutes on each side or until browned.

8. Top with sliced spring onions and enjoy.

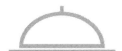

Courgette Fritters

Makes 3 servings

Prep time: 15 minutes | Cook time: 15 minutes | Total: 30 minutes

NET CARBS: 4.4G | PROTEIN: 13.5G | FIBRE: 2.7G | FAT: 23.9G
KCAL: 299

INGREDIENTS

- 2 courgettes
- 2 eggs
- 3 garlic cloves
- 1 spring onion
- 30g almond flour

- 50g grated parmesan cheese
- 30g shredded mozzarella
- 1 tbsp extra virgin olive oil
- 100g sour cream

INSTRUCTIONS

1. Grate the courgettes with a box grater until fully shredded. Finely slice the garlic and spring onion.

2. In a bowl, mix the shredded courgette with salt.

3. To drain the courgette of water, wrap in a kitchen towel or place in a colander. Hold over the sink and squeeze or press down until all the water is drained.

4. Back in the bowl, whisk two eggs. Combine with the shredded courgette, garlic, spring onion, parmesan cheese, shredded mozzarella, and almond flour. Season with black pepper.

5. Add olive oil to a pan over medium-high heat. Scoop a heaping tablespoon of the courgette mixture into the pan. Using a spatula or spoon, flatten until no more than 1cm thick. Cook for 2-3 minutes on each side until golden.

6. Serve with sour cream as a dipping sauce.

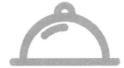

Desserts

Mini Keto Carrot Cakes

Makes 4 servings
Prep time: 10 minutes | Cook time: 10 minutes | Total: 20 minutes

NET CARBS: 12.4G | PROTEIN: 10.6G | FIBRE: 4.1G | FAT: 37.3G
KCAL: 426

INGREDIENTS

For the cake:

- 150g almond flour
- 80g shredded carrot
- 15g chopped walnuts
- 3 tbsps unsalted butter
- 2 large eggs
- 2 tbsps heavy whipping cream
- 2 tbsps powdered erythritol
- 2 tsps baking powder
- 1 tsp ground cinnamon

For the frosting:

- 50g full-fat cream cheese
- 2 tbsps butter
- 2 tsps powdered erythritol
- ½ tsp vanilla extract

INSTRUCTIONS

1. Preheat the oven to 180°C / 160°C (fan).
2. In a mixing bowl, combine the almond flour, cinnamon, baking powder, powdered erythritol, and chopped walnuts.
3. In a microwave safe bowl, heat the butter in the microwave for 30 seconds.
4. Pour the melted butter into the bowl of dry ingredients. Add the heavy whipping cream, shredded carrot, and eggs. Stir to fully combine.

5. Grease four small ramekins or oven-safe dessert bowls. Pour in the carrot cake mixture.
6. Bake for 10 minutes.
7. While the mini cakes are baking, combine the cream cheese and butter in a mixing bowl. Whisk vigorously or use a hand mixer to combine.
8. Once fluffy, add the powdered erythritol and vanilla extract. Mix well.
9. Turn the ramekins upside down and transfer the carrot cakes onto serving plates.
10. Divide the cream cheese frosting accordingly and top the cakes with an even layer.
11. Serve and enjoy.

Coconut Chia Pudding

Makes 2 servings
Prep time: 5 minutes | Total: 5 hours+

NET CARBS: | PROTEIN: 4.4G | FIBRE: 8.8G | FAT: 23.7G
KCAL: 377

INGREDIENTS

- 240ml coconut milk
- 70g chia seeds
- 10 raw blueberries

- ½ tsp vanilla extract
- 2 tsps erythritol*

INSTRUCTIONS

1. In two ramekins or other small-sized dessert bowls, combine the chia seeds and the coconut milk.
2. Stir thoroughly until all seeds are fully coated.
3. Cover and store in the refrigerator.
4. For best results, leave in the fridge overnight or at minimum 5 hours.
5. Serve with blueberries as a topping.

*To lower your intake of net carbs, 2 drops of stevia can be used as a substitute for erythritol. Please note, however, that stevia can add a touch of bitterness.

The 14 Days Keto Challenge

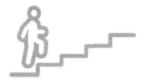

Breakfast: Sausage, Egg, and Veg Hash

Makes 2 servings

Prep time: 10 minutes | Cook time: 15 minutes | Total: 25 minutes

> NET CARBS: 4.5G | PROTEIN: 17.7G | FIBRE: 2.2G | FAT: 22.1G
> KCAL: 313

INGREDIENTS

- 4 sausages (Waitrose Free Range 97% Pork Sausages)
- 4 eggs
- 1 turnip
- 1 leek
- 1 spring onion
- 10g freshly chopped chives
- 1 tbsp butter

INSTRUCTIONS

1. Peel and dice the turnip. Finely slice the spring onion and chop the leek lengthways.

2. Heat butter in a pan at medium-high heat. Add the diced turnip and cook for 2-3 minutes, stirring occasionally.

3. Reduce the heat to medium-low heat. Add the sliced leeks and spring onion. Season with salt and pepper. Cook for 5 minutes together until the leeks are softened.

4. While the turnip and leeks are cooking, remove the sausage meat from their skins. Discard the skins.

5. Increase the heat on the pan to medium heat. Add the sausage meat and crumble into smaller pieces using a spatula. Cook for 4-5 minutes until all sausage meat is browned and cooked through.

6. Stir in all your freshly chopped chives, then remove from the pan.

7. Return the pan to medium-high heat with a dollop of butter.

8. Crack eggs into the pan and cook to your preference, about 2 minutes.

9. Add two fried eggs to each plate of turnip, sausage, and leek.

10. Serve and enjoy.

Lunch: Courgette Grilled Cheese (See page 40)

Dinner: Pork Loin with Cauliflower Mash (See page 51)

Breakfast: Mediterranean Breakfast Spread (See page 24)

Lunch: Cobb Salad

Makes 2 servings

Prep time: 10 minutes | Cook time: 3-5 minutes | Total: 15 minutes

NET CARBS: 5.1G | PROTEIN: 25.8G | FIBRE: 8.1G | FAT: 54.3G
KCAL: 645

INGREDIENTS

For the salad:

- ♦ 140g chopped lettuce or spinach
- ♦ 4 strips bacon
- ♦ 2 hard-boiled eggs
- ♦ 1 avocado
- ♦ ½ red onion

- ♦ 50g cherry tomatoes
- ♦ 30g blue cheese crumbles*
- ♦ 15g grated parmesan cheese
- ♦ 1 tbsp freshly chopped chives

For the dressing:

- ♦ 25g full-fat mayonnaise
- ♦ 25g sour cream

- ♦ 2 tsps red wine vinegar

INSTRUCTIONS

1. Cook the bacon strips over medium-low heat until browned and crispy. Let the bacon cool down while you continue with preparation.
2. Slice the red onions and chop the baby tomatoes in half.
3. Peel the avocado and remove the pit. Slice into thin wedges.

*Can be substituted for feta cheese.

4. Peel your hard-boiled eggs and slice into medium-sized wedges.

5. In a separate bowl, whisk together mayonnaise, sour cream, and red wine vinegar. Season well with salt and pepper.

6. Slice the cooked bacon strips into bite-sized pieces.

7. Begin assembling the salad by adding your chosen greens into a big serving bowl. Add the salad dressing, red onions, tomatoes, bacon, and blue cheese crumbles.

8. Top with boiled-egg wedges and avocado.

9. Serve with parmesan cheese and fresh chives.

Dinner: Chicken Rogan Josh (See page 55)

Breakfast: Breakfast Egg Bombs (See page 26)

Lunch: Chicken Butterhead Lettuce Wraps (See page 42)

Dinner: Coconut Curry Chicken with Cauliflower Rice

Makes 3 servings

Prep time: 15 minutes | Cook time: 25+ minutes | Total: 40+ minutes

> NET CARBS: 6.4G | PROTEIN: 30.8G | FIBRE: 4.9G | FAT: 52.4G
> KCAL: 854

INGREDIENTS

For the chicken curry:

- 320g boneless chicken thighs
- 300ml coconut cream
- 2 tbsps red curry paste
- 50g broccoli florets
- 1 white or yellow onion
- 2 garlic cloves
- 2 tbsp extra virgin olive oil or coconut oil
- 1 tsp ground ginger

For the cauliflower rice:

- 400g cauliflower
- 2 tbsps butter or coconut oil

INSTRUCTIONS

1. Prepare by finely chopping the onion and slicing the broccoli into bite-sized florets. Mince the garlic or finely chop.
2. Heat olive oil or coconut oil in a large pan over medium heat.

3. Cook the onions until browned for about 7 minutes, then remove from the pan and set aside.

4. Increase the heat on the pan to medium-high and add more of your chosen oil. Cook the chicken thighs for 2 minutes on each side until lightly golden on the outside. Use a spatula to press the chicken into the pan if necessary.

5. Add minced garlic, ground ginger, broccoli, coconut cream, and red powder paste to the pan. Season with salt and pepper.

6. Stir the mixture and bring to a boil.

7. Reduce the heat to medium-low and cover. Let the curry simmer for 15 minutes or until the chicken is cooked through.

8. While the curry simmers, use a food processor or box grater to rice your cauliflower. The stem can be included as well.

9. Optional: if your cauliflower looks wet, use a kitchen towel to remove any excess moisture.

10. In a separate pan, add butter or coconut oil and cook the cauliflower rice over medium heat for 8-10 minutes. Add salt. Cover while cooking to ensure that cauliflower stems get nicely softened.

11. Serve together.

Breakfast: Bacon, Eggs & Cabbage Hash Browns

Makes 2 servings

Prep time: 10 minutes | Cook time: 20 minutes | Total: 30 minutes

NET CARBS: 3.4G | PROTEIN: 44.1G | FIBRE: 3.4G | FAT: 41.2G
KCAL: 592

INGREDIENTS

For the bacon & eggs:

♦ 4 large eggs

♦ 4 slices bacon

For the cabbage hash browns:

♦ 2 large eggs

♦ ½ onion

♦ 220g shredded cabbage

♦ 2 tbsps extra virgin olive oil

♦ 1 garlic clove

♦ 50g full-fat sour cream

INSTRUCTIONS

1. Preheat the oven to 200°C / 180°C (fan).
2. Arrange the bacon slices on a baking tray in a single layer. No need to use oil.
3. Bake between 10-15 minutes depending on your personal preference.
4. While the bacon is in the oven, dice the onion and garlic.
5. In a bowl, whisk two eggs. Season with salt and pepper. Add the diced onion, garlic, and shredded cabbage. Stir to fully combine with the eggs.
6. Heat a pan with olive oil over medium-high heat.

7. Choose between four big hash patties or six smaller hash patties. Divide accordingly and scoop the cabbage mixture into the pan.
8. Cook until tender, about 3 minutes on each side. Use a spatula to flatten the patties.
9. Add a second pan with olive oil to the stove at medium-high heat. Break in the remaining eggs and fry to your preference, about 2-3 minutes.
10. Serve with sour cream on the side and enjoy.

Lunch: Caprese Stuffed Mushrooms (See page 37)
Dinner: Keto Hawaiian Pizza (See page 63)

Breakfast: Keto Croque Madame (See page 31)

Lunch: Walnut & Avocado Salad

Makes 4 servings

Prep time: 20 minutes | Cook time: 10 minutes | Total: 30 minutes

> NET CARBS: 5.8G | PROTEIN: 11.5G | FIBRE: 6.2G | FAT: 35.9G
> KCAL: 404

INGREDIENTS

For the salad:

- 1 Romaine lettuce head (600g)
- 50g chopped walnuts
- 50g feta cheese crumbles
- 25g grated parmesan cheese

- 2 courgettes
- 1 avocado
- 1 red onion
- 1 tbsp extra virgin olive oil

For the dressing:

- 3 tbsps extra virgin olive oil
- 2 tsps lemon juice

- 1 tsp apple cider vinegar

INSTRUCTIONS

1. Finely dice the red onion and quarter-slice the courgettes. Cut the avocado into bite-sized chunks about 1-2cm thick.

2. Wash the Romaine lettuce then blot dry with a kitchen towel. Cut off the root and remove any yellowing leaves. Slice into bite-sized pieces then add to a salad bowl with the diced onions.

3. Heat olive oil in a pan over medium heat. Add the courgette quarters to the pan. Season with salt and pepper. Cook for 8 minutes.

4. Add the chopped walnuts to the pan. Scatter grated parmesan cheese over the walnut and courgette mixture. Cook for another 2 minutes or until the courgette is lightly browned.

5. Take the courgette and walnuts off heat, and add to the bowl of Romaine lettuce and diced onions.

6. In a small bowl, combine the olive oil, lemon juice, and apple cider vinegar. Pour over the salad and toss so all the leaves are coated.

7. Top the salad with avocado chunks and feta cheese crumbles, then serve.

Dinner: Lemon Cream Salmon (See page 50)

| DAY 6 |

Breakfast: Tuna-Stuffed Avocado (See page 25)

Lunch: Watermelon & Prosciutto Salad (See page 39)

Dinner: Bunless Burgers

Makes 4 servings (1 each)

Prep time: 15 minutes | Cook time: 20 minutes | Total: 35 minutes

> NET CARBS: 5G | PROTEIN: 42G | FIBRE: 1.5G | FAT: 24.4G
> KCAL: 435

INGREDIENTS

For the burger:

- 450g ground beef
- 1 lettuce head
- 1 onion
- ½ tsp mustard
- 4 slices of any cheese
- 1 tbsp butter

For the sauce:

- 4 tbsps mayonnaise
- 2 tbsps tomato paste or sugar-free ketchup
- ¼ tsp white vinegar
- ½ tsp onion powder

INSTRUCTIONS

1. Whisk together the mayonnaise, tomato paste, white vinegar, and onion powder until it forms a smooth sauce. Cool in the fridge until your burgers are ready.

2. Prepare the veggie buns by cutting your lettuce head into quarters.

3. Chop the onion to your preference, either diced or into rings.

4. Separate the ground beef into 4 meat patties. Season with salt and pepper. Flatten to your desired thickness, but no more than 1cm.

5. Heat up a pan with butter to medium-low heat. Cook the onions until golden, about 8-10 minutes, then remove from the pan.

6. Place the meat patties on the pan. With a brush or spatula, top with a thin layer of mustard so they're lightly coated.

7. Cook the beef patties to your desired preference, but at least 2 minutes on each side.

8. Add a slice of cheese and tomato to each beef patty, then wrap in a swathe of lettuce. By hand or with a spoon, insert the onion into your bunless burger.

9. Serve with the chilled sauce.

Breakfast: Feta & Greens Scramble

Makes 2 servings

Prep time: 5 minutes | Cook time: 5 minutes | Total: 10 minutes

NET CARBS: 1.5G | PROTEIN: 21G | FIBRE: 2.6G | FAT: 22.5G
KCAL: 298

INGREDIENTS

- 120g spinach
- 50g feta cheese crumbles
- 10g grated parmesan cheese
- 4 large eggs
- 1 garlic clove
- 1 tbsp butter
- 100g cherry tomatoes (optional)

INSTRUCTIONS

1. Finely dice the garlic. In a bowl, whisk the eggs.
2. Heat a skillet with butter at medium heat. Add the spinach and garlic. Cook for 1-2 minutes until the spinach has wilted.
3. Pour the egg mixture into the pan. Allow the egg to set slightly before turning to scramble.
4. Add the parmesan cheese. Stir to mix and melt into the egg.
5. Transfer the scrambled eggs to plates and top with feta cheese crumbles.
6. Serve with halved cherry tomatoes on the side and enjoy.

Lunch: Cheesy Spinach & Tomato Pie (See page 48)

Dinner: Creamy White Chicken Chili (See page 65)

Breakfast: Spanish Baked Eggs (See page 29)

Lunch: Bacon Sushi

Makes 4 servings (4 each)

Prep time: 20 minutes | Cook time: 20 minutes | Total: 40 minutes

NET CARBS: 3.5G | PROTEIN: 12G | FIBRE: 4.1G | FAT: 45.6G
KCAL: 491

INGREDIENTS

- ♦ 120g full-fat cream cheese
- ♦ 8 slices bacon
- ♦ ½ cucumber
- ♦ 1 carrot
- ♦ 1 avocado

INSTRUCTIONS

1. Preheat the oven to 200°C / 180°C (fan).

2. While it heats up, cut the cucumber and carrot into thin slices, about 3-4cm in length so it fits perfectly in the bacon. Peel and pit the avocado, then chop into chunks of a similar length at 3-4cm.

3. Lay the strips of bacon onto a baking tray covered in parchment paper. Bake for 20 minutes, making sure to turn the rashers halfway through.

4. Dab the cooked bacon with a paper towel to remove some of the grease. Slice into even halves.

5. Arrange the sushi by placing a heaping teaspoon of cream cheese into each bacon half. Add a few slices of cucumber and carrot, and a chunk of avocado. Wrap the bacon. Repeat until all slices of bacon are filled.

6. Serve and enjoy.

Dinner: Eggplant Parmigiana (See page 53)

Breakfast: Almond Flour Waffles (See page 27)

Lunch: One-Pan Garlic Chicken & Broccoli (See page 36)

Dinner: Asian-Style Egg & Pork Bowl

Makes 3 servings

Prep time: 10 minutes | Cook time: 20 minutes | Total: 30 minutes

NET CARBS: 2.2G | PROTEIN: 33.8G | FIBRE: 2.6G | FAT: 46.3G
KCAL: 589

INGREDIENTS

- 460g ground pork
- 250g shredded cabbage
- 4 garlic cloves
- 3 large eggs
- 2 spring onions
- ½ tsp ground ginger
- 2 tbsps soy sauce
- 1 tbsp apple cider vinegar
- 1 tbsp sesame oil
- 1 tbsp extra virgin olive oil

INSTRUCTIONS

1. Mince the garlic and finely slice the spring onions.
2. In a small bowl, combine the soy sauce and apple cider vinegar.
3. Heat olive oil in a pan over medium heat. Add the ground pork and use your spatula to break it up into smaller pieces. Cook for 8 minutes or until fully cooked through.
4. Add the garlic, ginger, and sesame oil to the pan. Cook until fragrant for about 1-2 minutes, stirring occasionally to mix the ginger and garlic with the pork.

5. Add the shredded cabbage to the pan. Season with salt and pepper. Mix together and cook for 3-4 more minutes.

6. Pour the soy sauce and vinegar blend into the pan. Stir until combined with the pork and cabbage.

7. Move the contents of the pan into serving bowls.

8. Turn up the heat on the pan to medium-high. Add the rest of the olive oil and break an egg into the pan. Fry to your desired consistency, about 1-2 minutes. Repeat until all the eggs are fried.

9. Top the pork and cabbage bowls with one fried egg each.

10. Garnish with sliced spring onions and enjoy.

Breakfast: Stuffed Bell Peppers

Makes 2 servings

Prep time: 5 minutes | Cook time: 40 minutes | Total: 45 minutes

> NET CARBS: 8.4G | PROTEIN: 29G | FIBRE: 3.4G | FAT: 29.5G
> KCAL: 424

INGREDIENTS

- 120g shredded cheddar or mozzarella cheese
- 120g chopped tomatoes (half a can)
- 80g ground beef (or any meat substitute)

- 2 large yellow bell peppers
- ½ onion
- 2 tbsps chives
- 1 tbsp extra virgin olive oil

INSTRUCTIONS

1. Preheat the oven to 180°C / 160°C (fan).
2. Remove the stems and cores of the bell peppers. Slice them in half then dice the onion.
3. In a pan with olive oil over medium heat, cook the onions for 3 minutes.
4. Add the ground beef or meat substitute. Stir to combine with the onions and garlic. Cook for 7-8 minutes until browned.
5. Pour in the chopped tomatoes and roughly ¾ of the shredded cheese. Stir to combine. Season with salt and pepper. Allow to simmer for 3-4 minutes.

6. Fill the pepper halves with your meat filling. Top with the remaining shredded cheese and bake for 20-25 minutes until the peppers begin to brown.

Lunch: Club Salad (See page 47)

Dinner: Garlic & Mushroom Steak Bites (See page 57)

Breakfast: Feta & Mushroom Egg Muffins (See page 33)

Lunch: Parmesan Broccoli Soup

Makes 4 servings

Prep time: 10 minutes | Cook time: 30 minutes | Total: 40 minutes

> NET CARBS: 9G | PROTEIN: 16.5G | FIBRE: 5.6G | FAT: 29.5G
> KCAL: 383

INGREDIENTS

- 750g broccoli (3 medium heads)
- 120g grated parmesan cheese
- 200ml heavy whipping cream
- 200ml unsweetened almond milk
- 1 leek
- 1 tsp thyme
- 1 tbsp butter

INSTRUCTIONS

1. Remove the root of the leek and thinly slice. Chop the broccoli into bite-sized florets.
2. Heat a large pot with butter over medium heat.
3. Cook the leeks for 4-5 minutes until they start to golden.
4. Add the broccoli, heavy whipping cream and almond milk to the pot.
5. Season well with salt and pepper. Add the parmesan cheese and thyme.

6. Bring to a boil, then cover and reduce to low heat.

7. Allow to simmer for 15-18 minutes until the soup has thickened.

8. Stir and serve.

Dinner: Lamb, Tomato & Coconut Curry (See page 58)

Breakfast: Keto Smoothie Bowl (See page 28)

Lunch: Salmon Sushi Rolls (See page 44)

Dinner: Keto Shepherd's Pie

Makes 4 servings

Prep time: 10 minutes | Cook time: 50 minutes | Total: 1 hour

NET CARBS: 6G | PROTEIN: 77.7G | FIBRE: 7.5G | FAT: 32.8G
KCAL: 683

INGREDIENTS

- 900g ground lamb
- 120g grated cheddar or parmesan cheese
- 60g sour cream
- 55ml red wine vinegar
- 3 garlic cloves
- 2 tbsps coconut flour
- 2 tbsps butter
- 1 medium cauliflower
- 1 onion
- 1 tbsp thyme
- 1 tsp oregano (optional)

INSTRUCTIONS

1. Finely dice the onion and mince the garlic. Chop the cauliflower into small florets. The smaller the pieces of cauliflower, the creamier the cauliflower mash will be.

2. Bring a pot of water to boil, then add the cauliflower florets with a generous sprinkling of salt. Boil for 10 minutes or until the cauliflower is tender.

3. Add butter and half of the minced garlic to the same pot. Cook at medium-high heat until the garlic is fragrant, about 45 seconds to 1 minute.

4. Puree the garlic and cauliflower in a food processor until smooth or use a hand-held masher.

5. Return the cauliflower and garlic blend to the pot. Add sour cream, salt, pepper, and most of the shredded cheese. Stir until fully combined.

6. Heat a pan at medium heat. Add the ground lamb and red wine vinegar. Season with salt, pepper, and thyme, then cook for about 9-10 minutes or until the lamb is browned.

7. Preheat the oven to 200°C / 180°C (fan).

8. When the lamb is cooked through, create an even layer at the bottom of an oven-safe casserole dish.

9. In the same pan used for the lamb, cook the diced onion for 3-4 minutes. Add the coconut flour and remainder of the minced garlic to the pan and cook for an additional minute or until fragrant.

10. Pour the onion and garlic mixture over the ground lamb.

11. Scoop out the cauliflower blend, creating an even layer on top of the meat. Sprinkle the remainder of the shredded cheese on top.

12. Bake for 25 minutes or until the cauliflower mash appears golden.

13. Serve as is or with oregano.

Breakfast: Cloud Eggs & Cheesy Ham

Makes 6 servings

Prep time: 15 minutes | Cook time: 10 minutes | Total: 25 minutes

NET CARBS: 1.5G | PROTEIN: 23.3G | FIBRE: 0.4G | FAT: 20.2G
KCAL: 284

INGREDIENTS

- 6 large eggs
- 6 slices of deli ham
- 6 slices of Swiss or cheddar cheese
- 100g grated parmesan cheese
- 1 tsp chives
- ½ tsp salt

INSTRUCTIONS

1. Preheat the oven to 230°C / 210°C (fan).
2. Separate the egg whites from the egg yolks,* putting the whites into a separate mixing bowl that has no trace of water or grease in it. Do not discard the yolks but set them aside for later.
3. Beat the egg whites until soft peaks begin to form. Use a whisk or electric mixer, but keep in mind this can take up to 5 minutes with a whisk.
4. Add the salt and parmesan cheese to the whisked egg whites. Season with pepper. Stir once or twice to combine.
5. On a baking tray, divide the egg whites into six separate mounds.
6. Use a spoon to create a small hole or well in the center of each mound.
7. Bake for 5 minutes. Keep the oven on after you remove the tray.

*In order for step 3 to be successful, it's important that there is absolutely no yolk in the egg whites after you separate them.

8. Add one egg yolk to each mound of egg whites, placing it carefully into the well you made with your spoon. Bake for an additional 3 minutes.

9. Meanwhile, arrange the ham and cheese slices. Place one slice of ham on each plate, then layer a cheese slice on top of each.

10. Serve one cloud egg on top of each ham and cheese stack. Enjoy.

Lunch: Garlic Butter Prawns (See page 46)

Dinner: Alfredo Courgetti Noodles (See page 60)

Breakfast: Herb & Prawn Omelette (See page 34)

Lunch: Avocado Egg Salad

Makes 2 servings

Prep time: 10 minutes | Total: 10 minutes

NET CARBS: 7.6G | PROTEIN: 18.5G | FIBRE: 8.9G | FAT: 34.2G
KCAL: 432

INGREDIENTS

- ◆ 30g grated parmesan cheese
- ◆ 4 hard-boiled eggs
- ◆ 1 avocado
- ◆ 2 limes
- ◆ 2 tbsps chopped red onion
- ◆ 1 tbsp mayonnaise
- ◆ 1 tbsp chopped chives

INSTRUCTIONS

1. Scoop out the avocado flesh into a bowl. Add mayonnaise, chopped chives, and chopped onions.
2. Squeeze the juice of one and a half limes into the bowl, saving half a lime for garnish. Season with salt and pepper.
3. Stir to fully combine.
4. Add the hard-boiled eggs to the bowl and gently fold them into the mixture. They should be just barely combined but not too mixed in.
5. Transfer the avocado and egg salad into serving bowls.

6. Top with grated parmesan cheese.

7. Serve with a lime wedge garnish for each bowl.

Dinner: Chicken & Broccoli Casserole (See page 61)

Disclaimer

This book contains opinions and ideas of the author and is meant to teach the reader informative and helpful knowledge while due care should be taken by the user in the application of the information provided. The instructions and strategies are possibly not right for every reader and there is no guarantee that they work for everyone. Using this book and implementing the information/ recipes therein contained is explicitly your own responsibility and risk. This work with all its contents, does not guarantee correctness, completion, quality or correctness of the provided information. Misinformation or misprints cannot be completely eliminated.

Printed in Great Britain
by Amazon

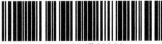